Essential Oils Horrible Mistakes:

25 Mistakes That Will Affect and Harm Your Health!

I0455747

Table of content

Introduction

I wish to thank and congratulate you for downloading "Essential Oils Horrible Mistakes: 25 Mistakes that Will Affect and Harm Your Health!" In this book, you will learn about many different types of applications of essential oils that should be avoided. By learning of these it will help to prepare you to make sure that you use safety and caution when using any essential oil. When you read about some of the horrible things that others had to suffer through due to applying or misusing essential oils, you will think twice before you begin to use essential oils.

Learning through other's mistakes will certainly help you when it comes to using essential oils safely. When you are aware of all the different unsafe applications, you will know to avoid them. Instead, you will go to the proper qualified individuals such as an aromatherapist to ask proper advice on any essential oils that you are interested in using. One of the biggest mistakes people make when it comes to using essential oils is that they simply do not do their homework and research. They do not bother to find out from reliable sources the proper and safe use of the essential oil they want to try. This is when many will misuse an essential oil and end up with some kind of bad reaction to the essential oil they have misused. I hope the collection of misuses of essential oils in this book will help you to learn what uses or applications to avoid.

Chapter 1. What Are Essential Oils?

Essential oils are usually obtained through a distillation process and having the characteristic fragrance of the plant from which it is extracted. I am sure you have enjoyd the smell of fresh flowers many times throughout your life. Volatile aromatic compounds are found in bark, stems, seeds, roots, flowers of plants. They offer us both, powerful and beautiful fragrances, filling our senses. It is the essential oils that are responsible for giving plants their individual unique smells. Essential oils also help to protect the plant and are an essential part in the plant pollination process. For thousands of years humans have included essential oils in various forms of health-care practices, beauty treatment, as well as food preparation.

The small organic molecules, known as volatile aromatic compounds change quickly from their liquid or solid form into a gas form when exposed to room temperature. They are referred to as volatile based on them being able to change form quickly. The first thing you will be aware when you open a bottle contianing essential oil is the strong and powerful scent that is released from within the bottle. The combination of physical and chemical properties of the volatile aromatic compounds compose the essential oils allowing them to travel fast through the air. They directly interact with the olfactory sensors in our nose's. These qualities make the use of essential oils in aromatherapy ideal. The use of these compounds is used to help promote overall health and wellness in both mind and body. The types of volatile aromatic compounds present in an essential oils help to determine what type of benefits that particular essential oil will offer.

There are thousands of varieties of volatile aromatic compounds to choose from. Essential oils differ from one plant species to the next. The ratio of aromatic constituents found in essential oils helps to determine the kinds of benefits that you can gain from an essential oil.

The length of time of distillation process as well as the method used, geographical location and season can all be contributing factors that will affect the composition of the essential oil. The weather can certianly influence every step of the production process; being a vital component when determining the overall quality of the essential oil.

There are a wide assortment of applications of essential oils from physical wellness to emotional applications. Essential oils can be applied as a single essential oil or they might be a blend of essential oils depending on what the desired benefit is and what is needed to recieve that benefit from the essential oils. Harm to one's health can occur when essential oils are not properly applied!

There is a good reason why essential oils are so popular. Mainly due to the fact that are pharmaceutical grade natural remedies with incredible power. However, with great power comes great responsibility. I love using essential oils, but when I use them I dilute them in my natural cleaning recipes, I also use them aromatically and therapeutically.

I make sure never to overuse essential oils due to their incredible power and being so concentrated.

Did you know it takes:

- 255 pounds of peppermint leaves to make one pound of peppermint essential oil
- 150 pounds of lavender flowers are needed to make one pound of lavender essential oil
- it takes thousands of pounds of roses to make 1 pound of rose essential oil

The properties of essential oils are very concentrated. You can can the same qualities from a very small amount of essential oil that you would gain from many cups of herbal tea from the same plant. For example, you would need to drink 25 cups of peppermint tea to gain the same benefits that you would get from 1 drop of peppermint essential oil. You must be careful when using essential oils. Use the proper amounts that are safe to use.

Essential Oils on the Skin

I love using beauty recipes that include essential oils, such as herbal face oil, but in diluted amounts. In most cases, you should not use undiluted essential oils on your skin. Essential oils have a very small molecular size, they easily penetrate the skin and enter the blood stream.

When it comes to using essential oils, a general rule of thumb is that they should be diluted in a carrier oil such as coconut oil or almond oil in a 3-5% solution. If you use 3-5 drops of essential oil mix it with 1 teaspoon of a carrier oil.

An allergic reaction or irritation can occur when essential oils are used undiluted on the skin. Some people may end up with a permanent sensitivity to a certain oil after using it undiluted on broken skin. Essential oils such as rose, chamomile and lavender are safe to use undiluted on skin. I personally still prefer to dilute all essential oils that I use. It is better to be safe than sorry.

I like to do a test on a small patch of skin on my arm with diluted essential oil that I want to use, before I apply it all over my body. I would say that the bottom line is to make sure that you do your research on any essential oil you plan on using, especially be cautious when using undiluted on your skin. I would suggest that you play it safe and dilute all essential oils that you use.

Common uses for essential oils
Health Support:

Due to their healing properties, essebtial oils have been used by humans for thousands of years. The naturally occurring chemical compounds found in essential oils help to mitigate ailments of all kinds when properly applied.

Managing mood:

Essential oils can be used to help us to manage our moods and emotions, helping us achieve balance in our lives. When essential oils are applied through the use of a diffuser they will directly affect the limbic system. Within the limbic system there is housed several structures in our brains that help influence our mood and emotions. Bio-chemicals are what cause us to experience emotions, as they are released into our system. The interaction that occurs between essential oils and these biochemical compounds can help to shift our mood. For example, have you ever walked into your home and there was a scent in the air of fresh baked cookies?—this scent may bring you back to a happy time in your life when your mother used to bake cookies for you as a child. Scents do have a very powerful effect on us both psychologically and physically.

Carrier oils:

Carrier oils are the fatty parts of plant-derived oils that are used to carry the essential oils to the skin in order to apply their benefits safely by diluting them. You will also gain nutritional benefits from carrier oils. Some of the more common carrier oils used with essential oils are:

Olive Oil: High in vitamin E and K, reduces fine lines and wrinkles.

Macadamia Nut Oil: It has one-to-one ration of omega-3 to omega-6 fatty acids, rich in phytochemicals, high in oleic acid and magnesium.

Sweet Almond Oil: Antioxidant, anti-inflammatory, rich in magnesium and vitamins A, B, E.

Grapeseed Oil: Antioxidant, anti-inflammatory rich in linoleic acid and vitamin E.

Jojoba Oil: Anti-inflammatory, astringent, and helps to balance sebum production in the skin.

Coconut Oil: Antimicrobial, anti-fungal, and a medium chain oil that can be used for food preparation as well as body care. It also contains vitamins E and K.

Application of Essential Oils:

Topically:

Some oils can be used neat or without a carrier oil such as lavender essential oil. Most essential oils do need to be in a carrier oil for an effective and safe application.

Aromatically:

Diffusing: Add essential oils to your diffuser according the manufacturers instructions.

Spritzing: Add 10-12 drops essential oil in a glass bottle filled with alcohol, shake well and spritz around the room, giving the room a boost in pleasant scent.

Steaming: Add 3-6 drops essential oil to hot water for steam diffusing.

Internally:

There are certain therapeutic essential oils that may be taken internally, in very tiny quantities and as directed. It is very important before using that you do your research.

Information is relayed to our brains when our nasal cavity senses detect the presence of chemicals in our environment, such as essential oils. .When the vaporized chemicals reach our nostrils, they dissolve in the mucus lying just under the surface of where our specialized receptor cells are located. These receptor cells detect and identify the odor and send the message to the limbic section of the brain.

This is an oversimplified explanation of how our sense of smell works. However, learning how to understand this fundamental element will help us to see why essential oils have such a strong and powerful impact on our physical, mental and emotional state.

We have not been able to pin point exactly when man discovered the significant value essential oils play in helping to enhance our quality of life. However, using them has been common practice in many civilizations around the world for thousands of years. If you are not familiar with essential oils and their uses, the thought of using smells, and scents, for healing may seem somewhat odd to you. However, with this been said, science has proven over the years that our olfactory systems carry a powerful punch when it comes to our health and mental state.

The limbic system is the area of our brian's that is responsible for identifying smells. This is the area that is connected to our central nervous system and the very seat of our motivations, emotions and our memory. That is why you could be walking along and get a whiff of a certain scent that sends you back in time to memory that you connect that particular smell to. It is largely for this reason that essential oils have played an important part in our lives. Essential oils have been used in our diets, cosmetics and even to help us to connect to our more spiritual being.

Chapter 2. Photosensitivity of Certain Essential Oils

When using citrus oils, I would exercise caution, because they can make your skin more sensitive to the sun. Citrus oils have certain constituents that can make the skin more sensitive to UV light and can lead to blistering, burning and discoloration of the skin much easier from just having minor sun exposure. The level of risk on developing photosensitivity or phototoxicity will largely depend on the way the essential oi was distilled, essential oils that are considered photosensitive are: grapefruit, bergamot, lemon, lime and orange.

Internal Use of Essential Oils

This is a controversial point, as many essential oils are not safe for internal use and others should be used with extreme caution. Since essential oils are equivalent of 10-50 cups of herbal tea (depending on the herb) or 20x the recommended dose of an herbal tincture of the same herb, they should only be taken internally in situations where they are needed and with extreme caution and care (under the guidance of a trained professional).

Essential oils are very potent plant compounds that can have a very dramatic effect on the human body. There are many online sources that are pushing the antibacterial, antiviral, and antifungal properties of essential oils. Your gut is something that is teeming with many types of bacteria.

Constantly there is new research emerging about our extremely diverse gut microbiomes, but we still do not completely understand them yet. We are aware that our gut health can affect other aspects of our overall health, imbalances in our gut can cause problems in other areas of our bodies such as skin, and the brain. The effects that essential oils has on gut bacteria has not really been studied in-depth. However, using essential oils with their antibacterial properties may be killing many types of bacteria in our guts, including beneficial and necessary bacteria. It is also been suggested that essential oils may be an effective alternative to antibiotics.

Antibiotics can be life-saving and necessary in some cases, but they should not be used regularly, or without the oversight of a medical professional. We should also exercise the same caution when using essential oils internally. In some cases, the benefits of essential oils (taken internally) can be obtained by using the herb itself (fresh or dried) in a tincture or tea of that herb.

Many essential oils are considered as safe to use for food or cosmetic use. However, many essential oils have not been studied, especially in concentrated internal amounts. Things such as baking soda, vinegar, and salt are also given this status. This does not mean that they should be consumed in copious amounts—do your research first!

Essential Oils During Pregnancy & Nursing

Extreme care should be taken when taking essential oils during pregnancy or nursing, due to the affect they have on hormones, gut bacteria and other aspects of health. There has been evidence that essential oils can cross the placenta and get to the baby. I am not saying you should not use them during pregnancy, but I would caution you to take extreme care during this time in using them. I would not take essential oils during pregnancy or nursing. During these times, I stick to aromatherapy.

I would first check with a professional and use caution with any herbs during pregnancy. Even essential oils that have been said to be safe, could be harmful to certain women, it is thought that essential oils can also cause dangerous hormone imbalances during pregnancy.

Oils Considered Not Safe During Pregnancy

Angelica, aniseed, basil, black pepper, cinnamon, camphor, clary sage, chamomile, fennel, ginger, jasmine, juniper, mustard, marjoram, rosemary, sage, thyme, oregano, peppermint, nutmeg, and wintergreen. I would check with your doctor or midwife before using any essential oils during pregnancy. Peppermint essential oil may decrease milk supply while nursing.

Use on Babies and Children

One of the things that concerns me the most is recommendations for essential oil use that I see online. I believe that essential oils should never be given to children internally or undiluted on the skin. In general oils such as chamomile, lavender, lemon and frankincense are considered safe for diluted use on children, but I would suggest checking with your doctor first.

Some oils have even been known to cause seizures in children, extreme cause should be used. This type of reaction is very rare, and it was mainly with people that had a predisposed seizure condition.

You should avoid using eucalyptus, wintergreen, rosemary and peppermint around small children. These herbs contain cineole and menthol. These compounds could slow down breathing in very young children or those that suffer from respiratory problems. These oils warrant caution, even with aromatic use. I would not use these oils on or around small children.

Essential Oils in Plastics

You should never store essential oils in plastic containers, especially concentrated forms. Many essential oils can easily eat through plastics when they are undiluted, and even when diluted, they will also degrade plastics over time.

I make homemade cleaners using essential oils, I store them in glass bottles for this reason. This caution is also extended to other surfaces within your home. I accidently knocked over some wild orange essential oil onto a piece of antique furniture. I didn't noticed I had knocked the bottle over until the next day when I discovered that the oil had taken the finish and stained an area on top of the table. Be careful how you store any essential oils, especially citrus based oils, make sure to store them safe and securely when not using.

Chapter 3. 25 Other Ways You Should Not Use Essential Oils

1. **For Bath**—You should not drop essential oils directly into your bath before getting in. Essential oils do not mix very well with water so they won't really be diluted in your bath. Chances are the oils will stay on the surface of the water where they can then cling to your skin. This can lead to chemical burns and essential oil side effects!

2. **Do Not Soak Tampon in Essential Oil**—before inserting them into your vagina. A woman that was suffering from a yeast infection was advised by an essential oil company to soak a tampon in tea tree essential oil and then insert it and leave it in overnight. The woman awoke in excruciating pain and ended up in the hospital to find that she had suffered chemical burns inside her vagina, where 3 months after the incident her doctor told her she had vaginal scarring. So, never put essential oils of any kind in or around your vagina.

3. **Do not use photo-sensitizing essential oils before going sunbathing.** Photo-sensitizing oils such as grapefruit and bergamot, and most citrus oils can burn and damage your skin when they are exposed to sunlight. A woman had an aromatherapy bath with included bergamot essential oil. After the bath, she spent 30 minutes in a sunbed. The next two days the woman noticed that her skin was red and blistering in areas that were exposed to sunlight. This woman was admitted to the burns unit of a U.K. hospital with 70% superficial partial thickness burns. These are painful burns that will take up to two weeks to heal.

4. **Do not add essential oils to Neti pot.** A woman reported adding one or two drops of a popular blend of essential oils to eight ounces of saline solution. She used the mix in her Neti pot and was find until about 10 days later after the application, she noticed:

- Her jaw was hurting

- Her face was swollen

- Her sense of smell was diminished

When she was checked at an urgent care centre it was discovered that her sinuses were red, swollen, as well as the surrounding facial areas were swollen and inflamed, causing pain in her jaw. She was diagnosed with a sinus infection. She was treated with 2 different steroids that she received by injections along with a 10-day course of antibiotics. Two weeks later the woman was put on stronger antibiotics and a short course of oral steroids.

5. Keep essential oils away from your eyes. A man accidently got some oregano essential oils in his eye where he thought he was ready to die in pain, he spent the next hour trying to flush his eye out. He noted that he was lucky he was not left blind in that eye.

6. Do not use unfamiliar vials of essential oils. Do not apply essential oils to your body, especially if they are not yours. A woman found a vial of essential oils that claimed to relieve stress by applying the oils on temples, forehead and back of neck. It contained a combination of peppermint, frankincense and wintergreen essential oils. She applied the essential oils to areas mentioned, unfortunately she accidently got some in her eyes. The burning it caused to her eyes was almost unbearable.

7. Do not use essential oils for cold sores. A woman reported applying clove essential oil onto her cold sore, once per day for three days. Each time she applied it she felt a tingling and redness on the spot. However, the third morning she awoke to find her mouth covered in open, bleeding sores.

8. Do not spill essential oils on your clothes. Undiluted essential oils on your skin usually spells bad news for most. You can become sensitized or experience an allergic reaction to essential oils this way. And they can definitely burn your skin badly.

So, if you have any essential oil spills onto your clothing, you should change into new clothing and wash the oils out of the oil stained clothing. If you don't you could run the risk of getting redness in your skin, blisters, and other side effects.

9. You should not handle essential oils without protective clothing. When you are using essential oils, you should consider wearing gloves, googles and long pants and long-sleeved shirts. It is certainly better to be safe than sorry.

10. You should never use a whole lot of essential oils especially if they are undiluted. Essential oils are made up of several chemical compounds and when you lump a whole lot together, you can't be sure if they're going to interact well with your body.

11. Do not use essential oils as headache relief. A woman applied an essential oil company blend to her forehead, temples and back of neck. The blend contained lavender, wintergreen, peppermint, frankincense, cilantro, chamomile, basil, marjoram, and rosemary essential oils. She reported headache relief on the first day, but the following day she awoke to finding her skin was bumpy and itchy, and she had a red rash all over areas of skin she applied the essential oils that lasted for a week. After that anytime she would go into the sunlight it would reoccur, only in areas that were exposed to the sun. This severe sensitivity to the sun last 3 weeks.

12. You should not ingest a large amount of essential oils. If you ingest a lot of essential oils, especially multiple undiluted essential oils, this is not going to end well. I would suggest not ingesting essential oils at all! A woman reported ingesting about 35 drops of lemon essential oil. She took all of this over a 5-hour period. A few hours later she began to feel nausea, dry heaving, high blood pressure, dizziness, and a rapid heartbeat. Several days later she went to hospital. She was given an IV and saline.

13. You should not use undiluted essential oils on children. Before using essential oils on your children consider the following cases: There was case where a one month old was massaged with juniper essential oil. The baby reportedly began to suffer from convulsions, fluid in his lungs, renal failure and liver damage! Thankfully, after the child spent eleven days in ICU, he was released from hospital in good condition.

Another case was when an undiluted essential oil company blend that contained eucalyptus, lemon, peppermint, thyme, and Melissa essential oils was applied to the chest, behind the ears, and armpits of a two-year-old boy. The poor child experienced seizures, foaming at the mouth and then he stopped breathing. He was rushed to hospital, after treatment and washing of his skin, he was back to normal.

14. Check with your child's pediatrician before using diluted essential oils on them. There have been many studies that report essential oil poisonings in children. And they are not all accidental ingestion. Many kids have bad reactions to blends that their own parents massaged into their skins. This is why it is best to discuss this with your child's pediatrician first before using.

There was a case where a six-year old girl had hives. Her guardians applied liberal amounts of a home remedy containing eucalyptus essential oil. The child did not react well to the remedy. She began to experience slurred speech and muscle weakness before falling unconscious. Six hours later after the oil remedy was washed off the child her symptoms were resolved.

15. Do not add essential oils directly to your child's bath water. To use essential oils safely they must be diluted. If not you are putting your child at risk of a chemical burn. There was a case where a four-year old boy was in his bath, when essential oil was added to the bath with. The child had broken out in hives immediately, he was quickly removed from the bath and washed and rinsed up. The reaction stopped immediately.

16. You should not use essential oils on your pets. According to the ASPCA eucalyptus essential oil is toxic to dogs, cats and horses. If your pet ingests this oil, they will probably begin to salivate excessively, and begin to vomit and have diarrhea, depression and weakness. A study also showed that using too much tea tree essential oil on your pets can also cause them to suffer from depression, in-coordination and muscle tremors.

17. Do not use essential oils to cure Ebola. When the epidemic of Ebola was in full swing in 2014-2015, essential oil companies attempted to capitalize on the fears of people by suggesting that their essential oil products could cure this deadly virus. Companies were sent warning letters from the FDA of specific violations these companies were doing. The companies did retract their claims.

18. Do not use essential oils as a source of vitamins. There was an article that was published online claiming that the peppermint essential oil contained vitamins A and C. The truth is that there aren't any vitamins in essential oils—none of them!

19. Do your homework before using essential oils. Before you begin to use essential oils in a way that perhaps some salesperson told you to, do your research first on the essential oil before you use it. Sales people are not medical experts you are better to talk to an experienced aromatherapist about essential oils.

20. Don't use essential oils in a way some blog or video tells you to. Do not follow blogs or groups that are telling you to ingest essential oils. You should speak to your doctor and do patch testing before using essential oils.

Groups could be giving you recipes and have the dilution rates totally wrong, which could cause great damage to some poor unsuspecting person that decides to try their deadly recipes.

21. Do not use essential oils based on claims made by an essential oil company. You really need to do your homework, check with your doctor and do a patch test before using any essential oils. Essential oil companies have made false claims—such as the Ebola cure promise.

22. Just because essential oils are 100% natural does not mean they are safe to ingest or use. You need to understand that essential oils are very potent, be aware of the risks and use safety and proper usage techniques.

23. Do not use essential oils because you think they are a detox or will remove toxins. If you use essential oils and then break out in hives or have some bad reaction to the oils and the person that sold them to you tells you that you are just detoxing—to not deal with them again. This person does not know what they are talking about. Instead, you should be consulting your doctor. An allergic reaction to essential oils is not your body's way of detoxing.

24. Why you shouldn't use essential oils while on prescription medications. You could have a drug interaction when using essential oils with prescription medications. Always check with your doctor first before using any essential oils while on prescribed medications. A case in 2012 noted that aniseed essential oil could interact with central nervous system. As a result, using this oil and these types of drugs simultaneously should be avoided. There have been many other drugs that can interact with essential oils.

25. Do not use essential oils in your diffuser if you are allergic. If you use high concentrations of essential oils in a poorly-ventilated space you could trigger undesirable effects such as an allergic reaction in yourself or others. So, you should certainly be cautious and considerate when diffusing essential oils in public spaces such as at the office etc.

Conclusion

I hope that you will use the information in this book to guide you towards safe applications of essential oils. As like most things they will work well when they are used in a manner that they were meant to be used. I can push it enough that it is very important that you do your research on essential oils that you are planning on using. It is always best to be safe than sorry. Like with most things that could affect your health it is always best to discuss things with your doctor to make sure using essential oils is safe for you. I am sure you will find using them very beneficial as long as you use them in a safe and responsible manner.

I would like to thank you once again for downloading my book, your support of my work means a great deal to me. I would love to read a review of my book by you on Amazon!

FREE Bonus Reminder

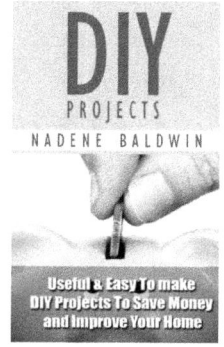

If you have not grabbed it yet, please go ahead and download your special bonus report *"DIY Projects. 13 Useful & Easy To Make DIY Projects To Save Money & Improve Your Home!"*

Simply Click the Button Below

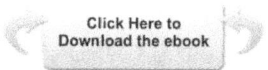

OR **Go to This Page**

http://diyhomecraft.com/free

BONUS #2: More Free & Discounted Books or Products

Do you want to receive more Free/Discounted Books or Products?

We have a mailing list where we send out our new Books or Products when they go free or with a discount on Amazon. Click on the link below to sign up for Free & Discount Book & Product Promotions.

=> Sign Up for Free & Discount Book & Product Promotions <=

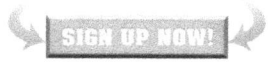

OR Go to this URL

http://zbit.ly/1WBb1Ek

www.ingramcontent.com/pod-product-compliance
Lightning Source LLC
Chambersburg PA
CBHW072024290526
45787CB00014B/1858